zeez: Step-by-Step Guide to Quality Sleep

ILIR HASKUKA

ISBN: 9781687032553

CONTENTS

ACKNOWLEDGMENTS

I am eternally grateful to my wife for always believing in me and supporting me throughout my life. She was in fact the first one to suggest that I should write a book to support the programme.

Knowing how passionate I am about psychology, my wife had introduced me to the Centre of Excellence online learning centre where I completed my Cognitive Behaviour Therapy (CBT) course.

The course was only the beginning of my learnings about CBT. I have learned just as much since, and I am still learning. Naturally, some of the notes and references from my learnings from the course work are woven into the programme and this book.

CHAPTER ONE:
The Book and the Programme

"A ruffled mind makes a restless pillow"
Charlotte Brontë

i. CONTENT

OVERVIEW

Sleep is a vital component of a healthy lifestyle, and it plays a crucial role in both physical and mental well-being. However, in today's fast-paced world, many people struggle to get the restful sleep they need. This programme is designed to provide you with practical tips and strategies for improving the quality of your sleep. Whether you have trouble falling asleep, staying asleep, or waking up feeling refreshed, this programme will help you identify the underlying causes of your sleep issues and provide you with effective solutions to help you achieve the restful, rejuvenating sleep you need.

This programme within the book is intended to provide practical and useful resources for anyone struggling with sleeplessness. We seek to present exceptional, noteworthy tips, tutorials, and resources that we believe people challenged with sleeplessness will appreciate.

All materials and resources shared in this book are from various credible sources and professionals from around the globe and from empirical evidence on the successes of Cognitive Behaviour Therapy for Insomnia (CBT-I). CBT-I is described in more details in Chapter 3, Sleep 101, CBT for Insomnia.

The programme was put together on the principles of an old proverb: " ... teach a man to fish ..." with the strongest mission to inspire everyone to go beyond overcoming sleeplessness, preventing sleeplessness and in the process learn about their own individual sleeping needs.

The programme puts high emphasis on the quality, comprehensiveness, and usefulness of each piece of material published in this book.

THE JOURNEY

I always enjoyed sharing my experiences and thoughts on the topic of sleep quality so the opportunity to share with a wider audience was very exciting to me.

I struggled with sleep deprivation in my early career when I was travelling excessively.
How can you tell if someone might be travelling extensively you might ask? Well, when on your way home, the customs officers ask you where you are coming from and you have to think for several seconds. Or when you wake up in the morning and wonder where you are. Or when the flight attendants recognise you by your name. Or when the customs officers ask you where do you live and then jokingly reply to you that you only have an address there. Or when you know your passport number by heart, and so on ...

Travelling had a huge impact on my sleep quality which in turn has had a direct impact on my job performance, as well as, when I got back home to my family.
So I learned a few techniques that really helped me ease some of my sleep related challenges and helped me adjust faster and better to new environments.
These new techniques that eventually developed into new habits helped me become more resilient for any future setbacks.

Initially, I started with asking a few colleagues that also travelled just as much or more. That followed with loads of reading and practising breathing techniques that required some mastering but worked really well.
Later on I learned some stretching techniques which helped a lot as well.
Many of these became habits that I still practise every day.

One other thing that helped with sleep that I started and followed religiously during all my travels was running. Yet I learned that running is not everyone's cup of tea hence there is little reference to this in the book.

In addition to learning a lot more about sleep and insomnia, the Cognitive Behaviour Therapy (CBT) course helped me to organise my thoughts and experiences enabling me to share these with others in this book.

HOW THE BOOK IS ORGANISED

The book is organised into four chapters:

Chapter 1: "ABOUT THE BOOK"
Has a few notes on how this book is organised, the programme
and model insights, how to get started, references and how to
provide feedback for us.

Chapter 2: "CREATING THE NEW SLEEP ROUTINE"
The core of the process and the programme of creating new
habits through CBT-I techniques to overcome sleep challenges.

Chapter 3: "SLEEP 101"
Covering general information on sleep and this chapter is
intended to help with education on sleep as well as help prevent
any future relapse or reoccurrence.

Chapter 4: "PRACTICAL GUIDANCE AND TOOLS"
Providing additional tools and resources to help with the journey.

Appendix pages:
We have provided some additional forms, templates, and
worksheets to help get you started and capture your progress.

ONLINE SUPPORT

The book is supported and accompanies an online application
programme titled "zeez", (https://www.zeez.online)

All material appearing in the book is also available through the
above mentioned online programme.

Although the online application came before the book, it evolved to provide ongoing support for the book, to engage with users and to continue to enrich the site with further tools and resources.

NOTES DATA PRIVACY (ONLINE SUPPORT)

The online application programme "zeez" is intentionally put together so minimum data is captured.

The only data that is captured is the user email address (anonymous by name) to help us manage, optimise the usage as well as make continuous improvements to the material and user experience.

No other data about the users is captured within the online application.
All the sleep data is designed to be tracked on external resources such as in the sleep diary, questionnaires, ... which are provided as external material and templates as downloads in the "MY TOOLS" section, as well as in the Appendix pages.

Additionally, we are providing a feedback loop which is optionally anonymous or the user can provide contact details for our response if that is expected.   Please see below.

FEEDBACK

In the spirit of continuous improvement, we would like to invite you to provide any feedback and comments you may have on making improvements.
Please visit https://www.zeez.online and share your thoughts with us.

ii. PROGRAMME OBJECTIVE

OVERVIEW

The programme is put together to help accomplish:
1. Improved sleep quality and quantity.
2. Reduced sleeplessness related daytime impairments.
3. Learn and practice techniques that will help with any future relapse or reoccurrence of sleeplessness.

The programme also works well when augmenting face-to-face care with a healthcare professional.
The programme is not intended to replace any sleeplessness related therapy for those who need it.

THE MODEL

The programme is broken down into time periods of the day that are in line with the circadian rhythm, the sleep drive as well as with the most impact on making progress in overcoming insomnia.

These time periods are described in more details in Chapter 2, "CREATING THE NEW SLEEP ROUTINE".

The five time periods are:

1. "Before Bedtime"
2. "Bedtime preparations"
3. "During Bedtime"
4. "After Bedtime"
5. "During Daytime"

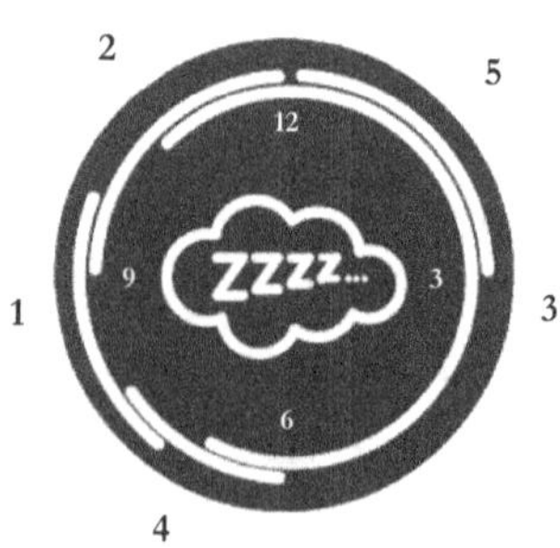

Each of the time periods are headlined with the three key principles of achieving results:
1. Goal - expected outcome.
2. Principle - the rationale, or the reason, or the purpose for the need to take action.
3. Actions - list of specific actions that include the key CBT-I components.

Each of these key CBT-I components are described in detail in the "SLEEP 101" section.

MNEMONICS

We are using simple Expression or Word Mnemonics to help remember the key activities for each of the five time periods of the day covered in the programme, such as R.E.S.T., R.E.L.A.X., S.L.E.E.P.Y., S.T.U.D.Y. and A.C.T.
For more details on each, please see Chapter 2.

BELIEFS

Much of the content in this book and the programme is focused on altering behaviour (habits) to make progress in overcoming sleeplessness.
It is worth mentioning the four most common unhelpful sleep-related cognitions and beliefs:

1. Unrealistic expectations about sleep requirements, for example: "I must get my 8 hours of sleep every night".
2. Faulty attributions about the causes of insomnia, for example:

"My insomnia is entirely due to a biochemical imbalance".
3. Excessive worry about sleep loss and amplification of its consequences, for example: "Insomnia will have serious consequences on my health".
4. Misconceptions about healthy sleep practices, for example: "If I only try harder, I'll eventually return to sleep". Some of these are deeply rooted beliefs and will require a longer-term approach, and in many cases may require professional therapy sessions.

WHO SHOULD NOT USE THIS PROGRAMME

Below is a list of recommendations for people that should not attempt to use this programme.
Please note that this list is not comprehensive or exhaustive in any way and there may be other conditions that may be best dealt with first, and separately, before starting any programmes such as this.

- If you have an acute illness such as infections. The programme should be used after full recovery.
- If you have been diagnosed with bipolar disorder.
- If you have been diagnosed with PTSD.
- If you are still in the process of alcohol abuse recovery.
- If you are using sedatives.

iii. GETTING STARTED

OVERVIEW

Let's face it: there is no magic pill! This programme (or any other similar programme) will only work with your determination and conviction to resolve challenges with sleep and make progress.

Probably the most surprising thing I came across whilst sharing the online application with people was that some people would say "I know all this" or "I know exactly what to do" and seemingly they would still continue their struggles with sleep with little willingness to even try.

We all know that this, and many other similar challenges, do require willingness, dedication, and persistence to make changes in our behaviour that supports overcoming these challenges. As boring as it may sound, we all know that to make favourable progress with anything that we do, the first step is to start!

And, this book is here to help you.

SETTING YOUR MISSION

One of the critical steps to getting started is working out how you will define a successful accomplishment. Setting a clear vision that matches your needs will help you make and track progress. Additionally, having a clear goal in mind will help you adjust and tweak the process as you move along.

What helps setting ourselves on a successful path is more often having clarity on a few things such as:

1. The what: what is it that you want to accomplish?
Your goal, direction, target, …
Some people aspire to sleep seven to eight hours a night, some focus on quality sleep, others have a specific daytime impairment (caused by sleeplessness) that they wish to remedy, and so on.

2. The why: why is this important to you?
Purpose gives us power or fuel to achieve our goals and objectives. Undoubtedly, there will be times when we confront key challenges on our path, and having a clear purpose will help overcome these and stay on the path.

3. The how: what is the actionable plan to achieve the goal, direction, target, …?
And this book (with the online application) aims to address this part.

It is necessary to highlight that initially some of the recommendations and actions will be counterintuitive and you must be ready to follow through.
 For example, your first goal will be to set your wake up time which has to be fixed and consistent every day of the week.
It is very important to adhere to this time.
You will start with the number of hours you currently sleep, which most certainly is not seven or eight if you are struggling with

sleep, and more likely may be something like five hours of sleep each night, or less.

So this then means that you will have to go to bed at 1 am if your wake up time goal is set to 6 am in the morning. And, it is extremely important that you stick to the same wake-up time, consistently and every day.

You will gradually increase your sleep time based on the feedback from your Sleep Diary (see below) and calculated Sleep Efficiency.

WHERE ARE YOU TODAY (setting the baseline)

Once committed to taking action, it is tremendously helpful for the future to "mark" where you started ("the stick in the sand"). This will additionally help you make progress and motivate you not only to keep going but also help avoid any future relapse.

To help with this, we have put together a Sleep Quality Questionnaire to help capture some of the information that is representative of your current challenges.

The questionnaire is available through the online programme https://www.zeez.online, "DOWNLOADS" section. Additionally, the questionnaire is also in Appendix 2.

And as mentioned before, in the interest of data privacy, we refrain from storing any such data within the application or anywhere online.

Also, we want to use every opportunity to discourage you from bringing your electronic devices to your bedroom.
Naturally, there are other forms, methodologies, and templates to

do so, and we just want to encourage you to choose one and use it.

TRACKING PROGRESS

Start keeping a Sleep Diary asap!

A Sleep Diary will help you identify what's keeping you awake.
A Sleep Diary will also help to progressively adjust the sleep efficiency targets to reach your optimum goals. Sometimes your sleep troubles are a result of bad sleep habits, for example, drinking too much caffeine before bedtime, not exercising or poor sleep hygiene.

The diary will help to highlight any patterns around when you are going to bed, when and how long do you typically wake-up during bedtime, when do you wake-up, and so on.
These patterns will help adjust times to increase the sleep efficiency and make progress.

A three-week sleep diary is available via the online programme https://www.zeez.online, "DOWNLOADS" section as well as Appendix A1 of this book.
Again, as mentioned before, in the interest of data privacy, we refrain from storing any such data within the application or anywhere online.

CHAPTER TWO:
Creating a New Sleep Routine

"It is not knowing what to do, it is doing what you know"
Tony Robbins

i. BEFORE BEDTIME
(early evening)

Typically between 19:00 to 22:00

THE GOAL
R.E.S.T. (wind down!)

THE PRINCIPLE
Before bedtime, it's essential to wind down and prepare both the body and mind for a restful night's sleep. Engaging in activities that promote relaxation is key.

One effective method is to immerse yourself in literature, whether it be a captivating book, an intriguing magazine, or an article focused on short stories. However, it's crucial to avoid getting too absorbed in strenuous reading or watching television, as this can stimulate the brain and hinder the transition to sleep. Instead, opt for lighter reading materials that won't overstimulate the mind.

Another beneficial practice is to engage in relaxed stretching and super-light exercises such as nighttime yoga. These gentle movements can help release tension accumulated throughout the day and signal to the body that it's time to unwind. It's important to note, though, that engaging in heavy exercises should be avoided at least two to three hours before bedtime, as they can invigorate the body rather than induce relaxation.

Additionally, if hunger strikes, opting for a light snack can help alleviate hunger pangs without causing discomfort during sleep. However, heavy meals should be avoided at least two hours before bedtime to prevent digestive issues that may disrupt sleep.

For those seeking a soothing beverage before bed, indulging in herbal teas known for their natural sedative effects, such as chamomile tea, can be incredibly calming. However, it's wise to steer clear of caffeine, nicotine, and alcohol, as they can interfere with sleep patterns and diminish the quality of rest.

By incorporating these winding-down activities into your bedtime routine, you can set the stage for a peaceful and rejuvenating night's sleep.

ACTIONS

R - Read: read a book, magazine or an article focused on short stories. Avoid getting immersed in strenuous reading or watching TV before bedtime.

E - Exercise: Practice a relaxed stretching and super-light exercises such as night-time yoga. Please take a look at some stretching exercises we have included in Appendix 4.
Avoid any heavy exercises at least two to three hours before bedtime.

S - Snack: if you are really hungry have a light snack.
Avoid heavy meals at least two hours before bedtime.

T - Tea-time: indulging in herbal teas that have a natural sedative effect can be both soothing and relaxing before bedtime, such as chamomile tea. Avoid caffeine, nicotine and alcohol.

ii. BEDTIME PREPARATIONS
(planned/scheduled bedtime)

Typically between 21:00 to 00:00

THE GOAL
R.E.L.A.X.

THE PRINCIPLE
Bedtime preparations are crucial for setting the stage for a restful night's sleep and ensuring that you enter a state of relaxation conducive to falling asleep easily.

Before heading to bed, it's important to assess whether you're truly ready to sleep. Ask yourself, "Am I ready to go to sleep?" If you don't feel sleepy, it's best to delay bedtime until you naturally feel tired. Avoid the temptation to bring activities or electronic devices into the bedroom, as they can stimulate the mind and interfere with your ability to unwind.

Additionally, resist the urge to sleep on a sofa or armchair, as these may not provide the proper support for quality sleep. Instead, reserve your bed for sleep and intimate activities only.

To facilitate a peaceful transition to sleep, it's essential to let go of any worries or concerns that may be weighing on your mind. If troubling thoughts arise just before bedtime, jot them down for consideration during designated "worry time" the following day. This practice can help prevent rumination and promote mental clarity before sleep. Address any tension in your body through relaxation techniques such as deep breathing exercises, meditation, gentle stretching, or nighttime yoga. These activities can help release physical and mental tension, preparing your body and mind for restorative sleep.

Furthermore, it's important to avoid clock-watching, as this can create anxiety about the passing time and disrupt your ability to relax. Wherever possible, remove all clocks from your bedroom or at least place them out of view.

If you find yourself awake for more than approximately 20 minutes (you can usually tell how long you have been awake), resist the urge to continuously check the time. Instead, leave the bedroom and engage in a quiet, non-stimulating activity until you feel sleepy again.

By following these bedtime preparations and guidelines, you can create an environment that promotes relaxation and sets the stage for a peaceful night's sleep.

ACTIONS

R - Ready: Ask yourself: "Am I ready to go to sleep?"
Simply do not go to bed unless you really are sleepy.

E - Ensure: Your bedroom is for sleeping only.
Avoid bringing any activities or devices into your bedroom.
Also, avoid sleeping on a sofa, or armchair or in any other room.

L - Let go: Let go of all your worries. Just note down any items or issues that pop-up just before bedtime and save these for the "worry time". There is more on this subject in Chapter 4, under the headline "Postpone your worries". Please take a look at the details provided.

A - Address any tension: Practice relaxation techniques such as breathing exercises, meditation, stretching, night-time yoga, and so on.
More details on all of these are provided in Chapter 4: PRACTICAL GUIDANCE AND TOOLS"

X - No clock watching: Remove all time/clock devices from your bedroom or at least from your view.
And, if you are awake for more than approximately 20 mins (remember: no clock-watching!), you must leave the bedroom.

iii. DURING BEDTIME
(waking up during bedtime)

Typically between 22:00 to 07:00

THE GOAL
S.L.E.E.P.Y (get sleepy!)

THE PRINCIPLE
During the winding down activities before bedtime, it's crucial to adopt a mindful approach to promote relaxation and prepare the body and mind for sleep.

One key aspect is to acknowledge that occasional awakenings during the night are normal and not a cause for alarm, reducing anxiety and unrealistic expectations.
Engaging in sedentary activities or tasks if waking up during bedtime can help minimize disruption to the sleep routine.

It's advisable to avoid embarking on significant endeavors such as cooking elaborate meals or undertaking extensive household chores, as these may stimulate the mind and delay the return to sleep.

Creating a conducive sleep environment involves minimizing exposure to bright lighting and noise, which can interfere with the body's natural circadian rhythms.
Embracing the notion that waking up during bedtime is part of the sleep process helps cultivate self-compassion and resilience in

dealing with sleep difficulties.

By prioritizing relaxation and minimizing stimuli, individuals can optimize their bedtime routine to facilitate restful and uninterrupted sleep,

ACTIONS

S - Sedentary: Take only sedentary (sitting down) activities or tasks when you wake up during your bedtime.

Avoid starting a big task such as cooking a full meal for the next day, or starting a major house clean up.

L - Lighting & Noise: Avoid exposure to both, bright lighting and noise.

E - Emphasise: It is important to note that it is OK to wake up during your bedtime when we are struggling to sleep and we must reassure ourselves that we are dealing with it.

E - Evolve: Take a note on when you woke up and how long you stayed awake and what helped you get back to sleep. Learning from these experiences will help you make progress in reducing the awake time as well as how many times we wake up during our bedtime.

P - Pacify & Persevere: Focus on calming down and getting sleepy by reading a book, magazine or an article focused on short stories.

And fight back getting immersed in heavy reading or watching long movies, especially thrillers. If TV relaxes you, then TV infomercials are probably best.

Y - Yawn: Go back to bed **only** when you can no longer stay awake.

Typically, yawning a few times is a good signal that you are ready.

iv. AFTER BEDTIME
(the first thing in the morning)

Typically between 06:00 to 08:30

THE GOAL
S.T.U.D.Y. (reflect and record!)

THE PRINCIPLE
After bedtime, winding down activities play a crucial role in preparing the mind and body for a restful night's sleep.

The first step involves taking notes from the previous night's sleep, an essential practice that shouldn't exceed five minutes. These notes are recorded in a sleep diary, a vital tool in addressing sleep-related challenges.
It's emphasized that the sleep diary is more of an art than a science, highlighting its subjective nature in tracking sleep patterns.
By tracking these patterns, adjustments can be made to optimize sleep efficiency and progress towards better sleep quality.

Consistency is key, with adherence to a fixed rise time every day, regardless of bedtime. The sleep diary serves as a reference point for identifying patterns that either support or hinder quality sleep habits. From there, individuals can devise a personalized sleep routine tailored to their needs, aiming for consistent, high-quality sleep.

Upon reaching set sleep quality targets, such as efficiency, it's important to take a moment to acknowledge and celebrate the achievement, reinforcing positive sleep habits and motivation for continued improvement.

ACTIONS

S - Stick to the rise time: You must ensure that you stick to the same fixed rise time, every day, regardless when you went to sleep.

T - Take notes: Note down the key information highlighted in your Sleep Diary from the night before. The sleep diary is included in Appendix 1. Alternatively, a three-week one-page Sleep Diary can be downloaded from the online application, https://www.zeez.online

U - Uncover: Learn about any patterns that support your habits for quality sleep as well as your habits that hinder a good quality sleep.

D - Determine: Work out what is the best sleep routine that helps you achieve a good quality sleep for you and how you will consistently aim to achieve that.

Y - Yield: When you reach your expected sleep quality target, such as the efficiency (see Chapter 3, "SLEEP 101"), it is important to take time and celebrate!

v. DURING DAYTIME
(ideally in the afternoon)

Typically between 12:00 to 15:00

THE GOAL
A.C.T. (tackle your worries!)

THE PRINCIPLE
During the daytime, winding down activities play a crucial role in preparing the mind for a restful night ahead.
In the midst of our bustling daily routines, finding moments to pause and reflect can often seem elusive.
However, allocating a specific time for this purpose, ideally in the afternoon, can prove immensely beneficial.
This designated period, often termed as "worry time," serves as an opportunity to review any lingering concerns or thoughts that may otherwise intrude upon the tranquility of bedtime.

It's essential to approach this time with a proactive mindset, understanding that not all issues can be resolved within the allocated timeframe.
Instead, the focus lies on devising actionable plans and scheduling dedicated slots to address them comprehensively.
By engaging in this practice consistently, individuals can mitigate the risk of nighttime anxieties and cultivate a sense of calmness before sleep. It's advisable to allot 10-15 minutes daily for this purpose, ensuring it becomes an integral part of one's routine.

Moreover, establishing a designated space outside the bedroom for "worry time" helps in delineating boundaries between relaxation and rumination.
Armed with a list of worries noted the night before, individuals can systematically address each concern, thereby fostering a sense of closure and mental clarity.

For further guidance on managing worries effectively, Appendix 3 "worry time tree" provides additional insights and recommendations. Thus, by incorporating these key winding down activities into daily life, individuals can nurture a conducive environment for restorative sleep and overall well-being.

ACTIONS

A - Action: Schedule 10-15 minutes of your time in your diary during the afternoon, every day.

C - Camp: Establish a place (not in the bedroom!) for "worry time".

T - Tackle: Go through your list of "worries" noted the night before and tackle and address each one of them and move on.

SUMMARY
(around the clock)

1. Before bedtime
Time: early evening - typically between 19:00 to 22:00
Goal: R.E.S.T. (wind down!)

2. Bedtime preparation
Time: planned/scheduled bedtime - typically between 21:00 to 00:00
Goal: R.E.L.A.X.

3. During bedtime
Time: waking up during sleep time - typically between 22:00 to 07:00
Goal: S.L.E.E.P.Y (get sleepy!)

4. After bedtime
Time: morning - typically between 06:00 to 08:30
Goal: S.T.U.D.Y. (reflect and record!)

5. During daytime
Time: afternoon - typically between 12:00 to 15:00
Goal: A.C.T. (tackle your worries!)

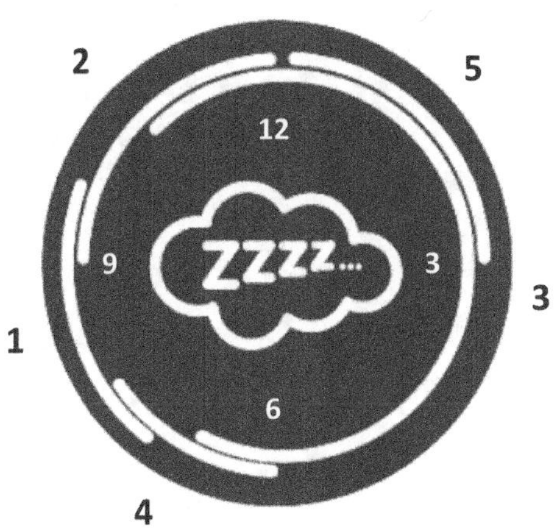

CHAPTER THREE:
Sleep 101

"You've got to be before you can do and do before you can have"
Zig Ziglar

i. GENERAL INFORMATION

Just like oxygen, food and water, sleep is one of our basic needs. It is just as important to our health as food and water.
Good sleep is good for the body and the mind. As we get the best out of every hour you sleep, we tend to get more out of every hour we wake up.

Some sleep scientists still do not seem to agree on the basic biological purpose of sleep.
Some do believe that during sleep, the human body restores and repairs cells and tissues that have been damaged while awake.
Other experts believe that sleep is essential for maintaining normal human metabolism.
And there seems to be little evidence that sleep is important for storing memories.

Despite all these differences, sleep experts generally agree that to function optimally, we all need consistently good sleep, and that sleep, both physically and emotionally, is vital to the overall wellbeing of our bodies.

These days our lifestyles are full of appointments, meetings, and extracurricular commitments, and as such we have an increased and more persistent sleep deficiencies in our society. Whilst some do hope that our body will adapt to sleep deprivation, science tells us otherwise. In response to sleep deficiencies, our bodies tend to respond in sluggishness, memory loss, poor judgment, and limited functionality.
Emotional and physical health can also be compromised, leading to high blood pressure, mood disorders and strained relationships.

Various factors contribute to sleep deficiencies, from stress and other lifestyle factors to health problems, physical problems or insomnia.

These days, sometimes even the terms "tired" and "sleepy" or "drowsy" seem to be used synonymously, even though they mean different things.

"Tired" can mean that the person has little energy, but does not necessarily have to sleep.

"Sleepy" generally refers to an actual need for sleep. If you think about your level of fatigue and drowsiness separately, you may be able to determine when you need sleep, rather than a general lack of energy. This can help you decide when to try to sleep and when to rest your body.

ii. SLEEP EFFICIENCY

Good quality sleep is all about the efficiency!

What is Sleep efficiency?
Sleep efficiency is the percentage of time spent asleep while in bed. It is calculated by dividing the amount of time spent asleep (in minutes) by the total amount of time in bed (in minutes).

A normal sleep efficiency is considered to be 85% or higher. Sleep efficiency calculations are taken from the sleep diary.

A typical sleep efficiency range is:
• normal sleep efficiency: 90%-95% (adult population).
• average sleep efficiency: 70%
• goal with this programme: 85%

The formula to calculate the sleep efficiency:
• time asleep / time in bed
• time asleep = time in bed - (time to fall asleep + time awake at night)

Example:
• Total sleep time=7 hours
• Subtract time it took to fall asleep=25 minutes
• Minus time awake = 25 minutes (5 minutes + 15 minutes +5 minutes)
• Total time asleep = 6 hours and 10 minutes (370 minutes)
• Now divide 370 minutes /420 minutes = 88%

The above formula will help make bedtime adjustments, based on sleep efficiency. For example:
if the sleep efficiency <85%, you can reduce time in bed by 15 minutes or, if sleep efficiency >90%, you can increase time in bed by 15 minutes and if in between, it is highly recommended to keep the time in bed the same.

iii. SLEEP REGULATORS

OVERVIEW

Two processes regulate sleep and wakefulness, the sleep drive and the circadian rhythm. Arousal also affects our ability to sleep.

SLEEP DRIVE

Our sleep drive is lowest in the morning and gradually increases as the day progresses. Sleeping gradually reduces our sleep drive as we "recharge our energy reserve", which is why napping close to bedtime (for example, dozing off while watching TV in the evening) can make it harder for us to fall asleep later. The longer the time that has elapsed since we last slept, the stronger is the sleep drive and the easier it will be to fall asleep. When the sleep drive is very strong we feel sleepy.

Homeostatic Drive

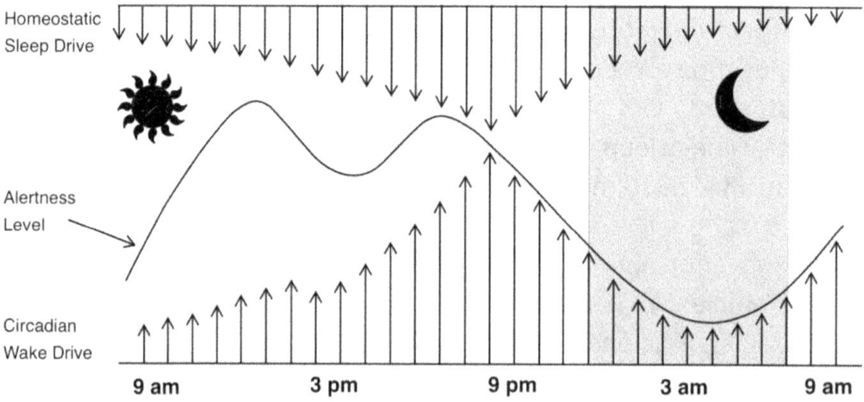

CIRCADIAN RHYTHM

People have powerful internal 'clocks' that affect their bodily functioning, including digestion, body temperature, and sleep/wake patterns. Most of these 'clocks' seem to work across roughly 24-hour periods. Irregular sleep schedules weaken our biological clocks, which is why it is particularly important to have a consistent wake up time.

Our body clocks use light signals to reset, so getting out of bed at the same time each day keeps the body clock ticking with a strong and regular beat, which supports good sleep.

Circadian Rhythm

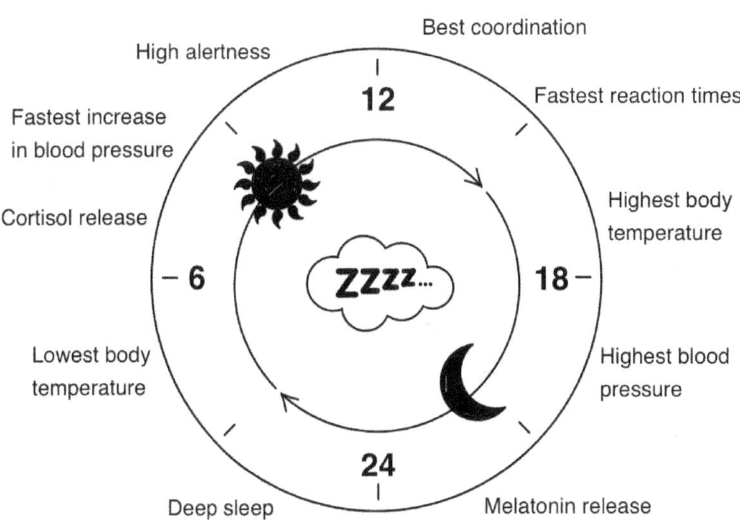

AROUSAL

Feeling "on guard" or anxious can mask sleepiness (strong sleep drive) and make sleep difficult. For example, when a sleep-deprived person is anxious before a job interview, this person generally does not feel sleepy during the interview, despite not getting enough sleep the night before. When the interview is over, and the person is relaxed, he or she may nod off while reading a magazine article because his or her strong sleep drive is no longer masked by anxiety.

This example demonstrates how the balance of sleep drive and arousal (such as a perceived threat, anxiety, active mind, or body tension) determines the likelihood of sleep at a given time. Common sources of arousal at bedtime include thinking about issues that have not been adequately resolved or addressed during the day, worrying about sleep, trying to remember what needs to be done the next day, anxious about the job interview and worrying about things not in one's control.

iv. SLEEP STAGES

OVERVIEW

Many research studies have shown that sleep is a process made up of two states: Rapid Eye Movement (REM sleep) and Non-Rapid Eye Movement (non REM) sleep. Non REM sleep is composed of several stages, and occupies about 75- 80% of the night's sleep of a "typical" young, healthy adult. The rest of the night's sleep is REM sleep.

Non-REM sleep consists of three sleep stages (N1, N2 and N3) that differ in their brain-wave activity patterns, perceived depth of sleep and in how much effort it takes to wake a person up.

Each sleep cycle lasts, on average, around 90 minutes.

N1 - "pre-sleep":
Typically around 5-10% of total sleep in adults.
People experience stage N1 sleep as very light. When awakened, many individuals think they have not been asleep. Nonetheless, stage N1 seems to be an essential part of normal sleep. People with insomnia and older adults spend more of their night's sleep in stage N1 than those without insomnia.

N2 - "light sleep":
Typically around 45 - 55% of total sleep in adults.
It is harder to wake a person from this stage and most people know they have been asleep.

N3 - "slow wave sleep":
Typically around 15 - 25% of total sleep in adults.
Brain activity during N3 sleep is also called slow-wave sleep because it is characterised by slow, distinctive waves called Delta waves. N3 is perceived as the deepest sleep and it is the hardest

stage to wake up from. People tend to have more stage N3 sleep on nights following prolonged wakefulness.

REM - "rapid eye movement":
Typically around 20 - 25% of total sleep in adults.
REM sleep is when most dreaming occurs. During REM sleep, bursts of rapid eye movements can be observed and heart and breathing rates become less regular. There is increased blood flow to the brain.
Interestingly, brain wave activities during REM sleep are a bit similar to those seen during wakefulness.
However, during REM sleep the body's skeletal muscles are in a state of relative paralysis which prevents people from 'acting out' their dreams.

Sleep Stages

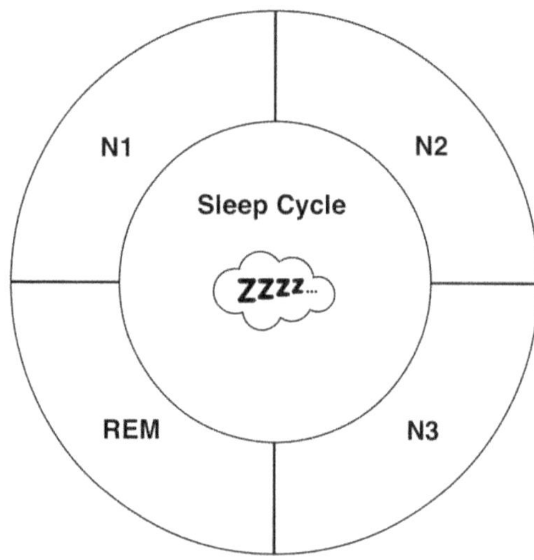

v. CBT FOR INSOMNIA

OVERVIEW

Cognitive Behavioural Therapy (CBT) is recognised as the best way to address insomnia because it does not use medicines and can, if done right and the patient sticks with it, lead to long-lasting elimination of insomnia. For many who have tried it, CBT has made a tremendous impact in providing lasting relief. CBT addresses a person's behaviour through providing education and establishing better sleep habits. Usually, patients attend several sessions (from 4 to 12) lasting about 30 minutes with a qualified sleep professional. Most commonly this is a psychologist with a special interest in insomnia, but nurse practitioners, physicians, psychiatrists, holistic therapists and others that direct patient care can also provide CBT if specially trained. In the process, misconceptions and misinformation about sleep in general are eliminated, and better sleep hygiene is developed.

CAUSES OF INSOMNIA - The '3 Ps' model

It would be great to think that insomnia had a single cause! It usually does not – The '3 Ps' model, designed to help people understand the development and persistence of health problems, was brought into research on poor sleep by Dr Art Spielman in the 1980s.

The three Ps stand for:
1. Predisposing
2. Precipitating
3. Perpetuating

1. Predisposing factors
A predisposition does not 'cause' a problem but may increase the likelihood of it occurring. When thinking about insomnia these

could include having a family history of poor sleep, generally being a 'worrier' or never having been a 'good sleeper', for example.

2. Precipitating factors

Another word for these could be 'triggers' and may include such things as lifestyle changes, a house move or promotion at work, the development of an illness or birth of a baby for example.

3. Perpetuating factors

These would cover any factors which might be seen to maintain or even exacerbate the problem e.g. heightened anxiety/arousal levels for or the development of depression which may represent barriers to recovery. It may also be the case that behaviours or coping strategies (e.g. napping during the day or spending excessive amounts of time in bed), developed and implemented over time are involved in the maintenance of insomnia.

Thus, insomnia could become learned over months and years, even though the initial stressor that may have been involved in its development has disappeared.

Sleep 3P's Model (Fig. a.)

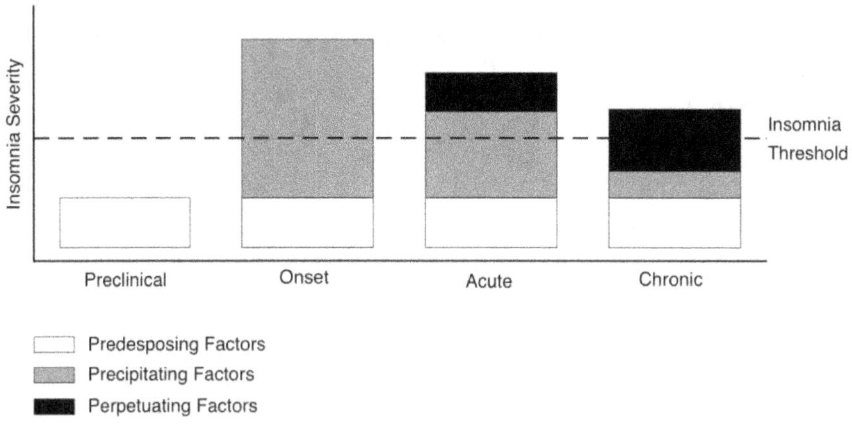

Sleep 3P's Model (Fig. b.)

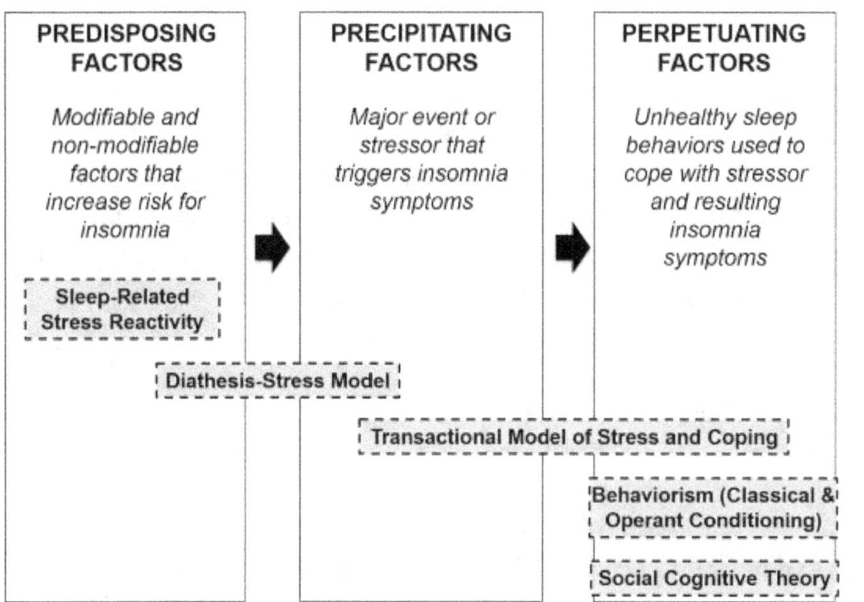

KEY CBT-I COMPONENTS

The key CBT for insomnia components are embedded in the list of actions for each time period of the day.

These include:
Stimulus control
Sleep restrictions
Relaxation techniques
Sleep hygiene

Each of these key components are described in more details below.

STIMULUS CONTROL

This set of instructions addresses conditioned arousal. It was developed by Richard Bootzin. They are designed to strengthen the bed as a cue for sleep and weaken it as a cue for wakefulness.

The key instructions are:

• **Establish a regular morning rise time.**
This will help strengthen the circadian clock regulating sleep and wakefulness. Ideally, bedtime should also be regular, but for people with insomnia it is impossible to actually fall asleep around the same time every night. When insomnia resolves, regular bedtime can further strengthen the circadian rhythm.

• **Go to bed only when sleepy.**
This will increase the probability that you will fall asleep quickly. It is important to distinguish between fatigue and sleepiness.
Fatigue is a state of low energy, physical or mental. Sleepiness is a state of having to struggle to stay awake. Dosing off while watching TV or as a passenger in a car involve sleepiness. People

with insomnia often feel tired but "wired" (i.e. not sleepy) at bedtime.

• If unable to fall asleep.
Either at the beginning or in the middle of the night, get out of bed and return to bed only when sleepy again.

• Avoid excessive napping during the day.
When facing sleep related challenges, we highly recommend to avoid an napping. However, when this is not realistic, a brief nap (15 to 30 minutes), taken approximately 7 to 9 hours after rise time, can be refreshing and is not likely to disturb nocturnal sleep.

SLEEP RESTRICTION

This procedure, developed by Arthur Spielman, is designed to eliminate prolonged middle of the night awakenings. It doesn't aim to restrict actual sleep time but rather to initially restrict the time spent in bed. Subsequent steps consist of gradually increasing the time spent in bed. The initial time in bed is usually the average nightly total sleep time over the last week. However, the time allowed in bed should not be less than 5.5 hours, even for people who sleep less than 5.5 hours per night. For example, consider a person who goes to bed at 11:00 p.m. and gets out of bed at 8:00 a.m. but sleeps on average only 6 hours per night. During the first step of this procedure this person will be in bed only 6 hours (e.g., 12:00 a.m. to 6:00 a.m.).

This sounds harsh but after a week or so there will be a marked decrease in time spent awake in the middle of the night. Usually people experience marked improvement in the quality of sleep after a week of restricted time in bed, but they also realise that they are not getting enough sleep. In this case, the next step is to gradually extend the time spent in bed by 15 to 30 minutes, as long as wakefulness in the middle of the night remains minimal.

Each new extension of the time in bed is followed for at least a week before progressing to the next extension. The decision as to when to extend the time in bed is based on the percent of the time slept relative to the time spent in bed. This is called sleep efficiency. If the average sleep efficiency is 85% or more, then the time in bed is extended. If it is below 80% then the time is bed is further restricted. Otherwise the time in bed remains unchanged.

There are several variants of this procedure, and the therapist chooses the one that best fits an individual patient. In all variants, the procedure continues until one reaches a point after which no further extension is necessary because the amount of sleep obtained is sufficient for optimal daytime function.

RELAXATION TECHNIQUES

The aim of relaxation techniques is to achieve physical and mental relaxation. They are meant to reduce physical tension and interrupt the thought processes that are affecting sleep. Studies show that people who have learned relaxation techniques sleep a bit longer at night. The main benefit of the relaxation techniques was being able to fall asleep somewhat more quickly. But these approaches don't help everyone.

There are different types of relaxation techniques:

• **Progressive muscle relaxation (or deep muscle relaxation)**
Progressive muscle relaxation (PMR) is a technique aimed at reducing muscle tension and promoting relaxation throughout the body. By systematically tensing and then releasing different muscle groups, PMR helps individuals become more attuned to the sensations of tension and relaxation, thereby enabling them

to consciously relax their muscles. This process not only aids in relieving physical tension but also promotes mental calmness and reduces stress levels. As a result, practicing PMR before bedtime can be highly beneficial for improving sleep quality. By incorporating PMR into a nightly routine, individuals can alleviate the physical and psychological factors that often interfere with sleep, such as muscle stiffness, racing thoughts, and overall stress. Ultimately, PMR can create a conducive environment for falling asleep faster, experiencing deeper sleep cycles, and waking up feeling more refreshed and rejuvenated.

• Autogenic training (AT)

Autogenic training involves focusing awareness on different parts of the body and consciously relaxing them. At an advanced level, even involuntary bodily functions like pulse and breathing can be influenced to achieve deep physical relaxation. Autogenic training is taught in courses.

• Biofeedback

This method helps you to feel how your body reacts to tensing and relaxing. It involves placing electrodes on your body to measure muscle tension, your pulse and brain activity. You can monitor these different measurements on a screen and see how muscle relaxation or thinking particular thoughts affects them. Biofeedback can be done at the doctor's or by using a portable biofeedback device at home once you've been instructed in how to use it.

• Visualisation

Another common type of relaxation training is imagery, where you visualise peaceful, pleasant scenes or imagine yourself breathing quietly, gently falling asleep and having a good night's sleep.

SLEEP HYGIENE

Sleep hygiene is a variety of different practices and habits that are necessary to have good nighttime sleep quality and full daytime alertness.

One of the most important sleep hygiene practices is to spend an appropriate amount of time asleep in bed, not too little or too excessive. Sleep needs vary across ages and are especially impacted by lifestyle and health. However, there are recommendations that can provide guidance on how much sleep you need generally.

Other good sleep hygiene practices include:

• Napping
Napping does not make up for inadequate nighttime sleep. Although a short nap of 20-30 minutes can help to improve mood, alertness and performance, when struggling with sleep, we recommend to avoid if and when possible.

• Stimulants
And when it comes to alcohol, moderation is key. While alcohol is well-known to help you fall asleep faster, too much close to bedtime can disrupt sleep in the second half of the night as the body begins to process the alcohol.

• Exercise
As little as 10 minutes of aerobic exercise, such as walking or cycling, can drastically improve nighttime sleep quality. For the best night's sleep, most people should avoid strenuous workouts close to bedtime. However, the effect of intense nighttime exercise on sleep differs from person to person, so find out what works best for you.

• Food
Heavy or rich foods, fatty or fried meals, spicy dishes, citrus fruits,

and carbonated drinks can trigger indigestion for some people. When this occurs close to bedtime, it can lead to painful heartburn that disrupts sleep.

• Exposure to natural light

This is particularly important for individuals who may not venture outside frequently. Exposure to sunlight during the day, as well as darkness at night, helps to maintain a healthy sleep-wake cycle.

• Establishing a sleep routine

Much of the practical approach to establishing a sleep routine is already covered in Chapter 2 "CREATING A NEW SLEEP ROUTINE". A regular sleep routine helps the body recognise that it is bedtime, such as, reading a book (short stories), or a magazine, or doing light stretches, practising breathing exercises, etc.

Please also refer to Chapter 4, "PRACTICAL GUIDANCE AND TOOLS" for more practical tools and approaches that support Sleep Hygiene items covered above.

CHAPTER FOUR:
Practical Guidance & Tools

"Sleep is the best meditation"
Dalai Lama

i. THE BEDROOM ENVIRONMENT

OVERVIEW

To get most of our effort in optimising our sleep we need to also look at our environment and areas we can improve. Below are some areas for consideration.

TEMPERATURE

Room temperature does have a huge impact on your sleep. Your body heat peaks in the evening and then drops to its lowest levels when you're asleep, so a cool 16-18°C (60-65°F) is thought to be an ideal temperature in a bedroom. Temperatures above this range are likely to cause restlessness, and on the other side, a colder room will make it difficult to drop off.
Younger children and elderly people may require a slightly warmer environment, so it is useful to invest in a room thermometer to keep track of temperatures.
It is also worth purchasing a range of suitable "seasonal" bedding depending on the season to better adjust and get more comfortable when it is cold, as will a hot water bottle or a good pair of bed socks for cold feet. Where and when possible (with safety and security in mind!), have windows open to maximise cool air circulation in the summer months.

COMFORT

Your bed is by far the most significant element of a good night's rest. It is near impossible to get a deep, effective sleep on an old, uncomfortable bed. Mattresses lacking comfort, space and support are likely to leave you waking tired and achy, and will also have a significant impact on your partner's sleep, too. Everyone is made differently, which is why different beds suit different bodies. You should select the best mattress for you, offering the correct support and comfort for your weight and build, and if someone else is going to be sharing the bed, spend extra time finding a mutually comfortable bed. When we are asleep it is recommended that we maintain a good posture; a mattress too soft will cause us to slouch, while one that's too firm can apply pressure to our hips and shoulders.

SOUND & LIGHTING

Other aspects of the bedroom environment are also the sound and the lighting we are exposed to in our bedrooms.
Please see below some notes and recommendations on both.

Sound:

Loud, sudden or repetitive noises can interrupt sleep. One of the best ways to combat this is with double glazing, as it muffles sounds from outside. You can also use foam ear plugs, which are particularly effective in the warmer months when you may leave a window open.
On the other side, whilst certain noises cause interrupted sleep, soft, steady sounds can be soothing. And many people find these types of sounds helpful and even essential to get a good night's sleep. For example, listening to 'white noise' sounds can help fall asleep and sleep more soundly. Others may prefer low familiar tones.

Lighting:

Lighting is also critical to our sleep as it can also trigger numerous chemical reactions in our bodies. For example, when we see light, our bodies assume it is time to wake up. When it is dark, we release melatonin, which relaxes the body and helps us to drift off.
So, it is no surprise that many more of us struggle to adjust to a new sleeping pattern during summertime seasons when it is light outside. And we notice this in particular when clocks change.

There's nothing worse than being rudely awoken by the early morning sun, so try blackout blinds or an eye mask.

Please remember to avoid having any clock devices at your sight level as having these clock devices tends to trigger
and elevate anxiety levels by constantly looking at the time.

And of course, the biggest challenge today is having mobile phones, tablets and computer screens in our bedrooms. These displays typically emit blue light, which suppresses melatonin.

SCENT & SMELL

Aromatherapy, the practice of using essential oils derived from plants for therapeutic purposes, has been recognized for its potential to promote relaxation and improve sleep quality. Research suggests that certain essential oils have sedative effects that can help alleviate insomnia and enhance sleep. One way aromatherapy aids sleep is through its ability to activate the limbic system, the part of the brain involved in emotions and memory, which can induce a state of relaxation conducive to falling asleep. Additionally, inhaling the aroma of essential oils can stimulate the release of neurotransmitters like serotonin and dopamine, which play a role in regulating mood and sleep-wake cycles. This dual action of calming the mind and body makes aromatherapy a popular natural remedy for sleep disturbances.

Numerous essential oils have been identified for their sleep-promoting properties. Lavender, perhaps the most well-known, has been extensively studied and shown to reduce anxiety and improve sleep quality. Other commonly used essential oils for sleep include chamomile, which has calming and sedative effects, and sandalwood, known for its ability to induce relaxation. Additionally, oils such as bergamot, ylang ylang, and cedarwood have been found to alleviate stress and promote feelings of tranquility, making them valuable additions to sleep-promoting blends. Citrus oils like sweet orange and bergamot can uplift mood and relieve tension, further contributing to a restful sleep environment.

For those seeking to incorporate essential oils into their sleep routine, it's essential to choose high-quality oils and use them safely. Recommendations for the best essential oils for sleep include lavender, chamomile, sandalwood, bergamot, ylang ylang, cedarwood, sweet orange, marjoram, valerian, frankincense, clary sage, and vetiver. To apply essential oils for sleep, a few drops can be added to a diffuser or mixed with a carrier oil and massaged onto the skin. Alternatively, a drop or two can be added to bedding, such as pillows or sheets, to create a calming atmosphere. It's important to dilute essential oils properly, as they can be potent and may cause irritation or adverse reactions if used undiluted. Additionally, some individuals may be sensitive to certain oils, so it's advisable to perform a patch test before widespread use.

While aromatherapy can be a valuable tool for improving sleep quality, it's crucial to exercise caution when using essential oils. Certain oils may interact with medications or exacerbate underlying health conditions, so individuals with medical concerns should consult with a healthcare professional before incorporating aromatherapy into their routine. Furthermore, pregnant women, young children, and pets may be more sensitive to certain essential oils and should use them sparingly or under the guidance of a qualified practitioner. Proper ventilation is also important when diffusing essential oils to prevent respiratory irritation. By following safety guidelines and choosing appropriate oils, aromatherapy can be a safe and effective way to promote relaxation and enhance sleep.

ii. BREATHING

OVERVIEW

Breathing plays a pivotal role in fostering quality sleep, acting as a bridge between wakefulness and restfulness. Deep, diaphragmatic breathing techniques such as belly breathing or paced breathing can induce a state of relaxation, effectively calming the nervous system and reducing stress levels. As individuals engage in intentional breathing exercises before bedtime, they signal to their bodies that it's time to unwind, allowing for a smoother transition into sleep. This rhythmic breathing pattern slows down the heart rate, lowers blood pressure, and releases tension stored in muscles, promoting a sense of tranquility conducive to falling asleep more easily.

Moreover, conscious breathing during sleep can enhance the overall quality of rest by optimizing oxygen intake and carbon dioxide release. Through steady, controlled breathing, the body maintains a balanced exchange of gases, ensuring that vital organs receive adequate oxygenation throughout the night. This optimized respiratory function supports various physiological processes during sleep, including tissue repair, muscle recovery, and cognitive consolidation. Additionally, deep breathing aids in regulating the body's natural circadian rhythms, synchronizing biological processes to promote more restorative sleep cycles. By harnessing the power of breath, individuals can cultivate a deeper and more rejuvenating sleep experience, waking up feeling refreshed and revitalized each morning.

VISUALISING BREATHING

Before starting, find a quiet place and sit in a comfortable laying down position.

With focus on breathing, as you inhale, envision the air traveling into your nose, through your entire body, and back out again. Imagine it traveling through all your muscles, all the way to your toes and fingers, before it comes back out again during your exhale.

Focusing on your breathing activates your parasympathetic system, encouraging it to calm down, relax, and lower your heart rate in preparation for sleep.

RELAXED BREATHING (the 3-6-9 method)

Before starting, find a quiet place and sit in a comfortable laying down position and place the tip of the tongue on the tissue right behind the top front teeth.

Follow the breathing pattern below:
Exhale through your mouth fully, to empty the lungs of air and making a "whoosh" sound as you do so.
Then breathe in quietly through the nose for three seconds, or to a count of three.
Hold your breath for a count of six seconds, or for the count of six.
Exhale forcefully but slowly through the mouth, pursing the lips and again making a "whoosh" sound, for nine seconds, or count of nine.
Repeat the cycle up to six times.

The ratio is very important here, so you may need to count faster until you can work your way up to slower breaths.

You may feel lightheaded after doing this for the first few times. Therefore, it is advisable to try this technique when sitting or lying down to prevent dizziness.

Please see the illustration below to help visualise the breathing pattern.

The 3-6-9 method

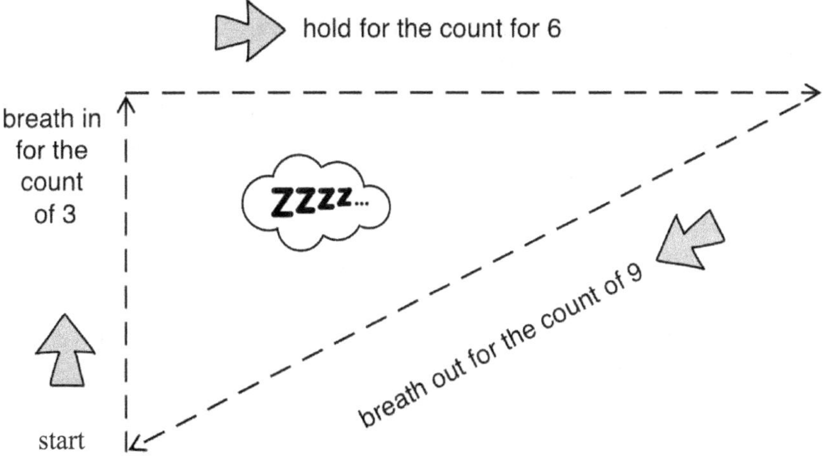

MEDITATIVE BREATHING

Before starting, find a quiet place and sit in a comfortable position.

It is most important to keep your back straight to prevent your mind from getting sleepy.

The first stage is to stop distractions and make your mind clearer. Close your eyes and focus on your breathing. Firstly, take a few deep breaths and then get back to breathing naturally, preferably through the nostrils.

Typically, at first, our mind will be very busy, and we might even feel that the meditation is making our mind busier; but in reality we are just becoming more aware of how busy our mind actually is. There will be a great temptation to follow the different thoughts as they arise, but we should resist this and remain focused on the sensation of the breath. If we discover that our mind has wandered and is following our thoughts, we should immediately return it to the breath. We should repeat this as many times as necessary until the mind settles on the breath. By keeping to this pattern you keep your mind focused on your breath instead of anxiety.

We recommend that you start with meditating for 10 minutes and then expand to longer as you get more comfortable with the practice .

DIAPHRAGMATIC BREATHING

Diaphragmatic breathing, also known as deep belly breathing or abdominal breathing, is a powerful technique that can significantly improve the quality of sleep. This method involves breathing deeply into the lungs, allowing the diaphragm to fully engage and expand the belly with each breath. By focusing on breathing from the diaphragm rather than shallowly from the chest, individuals can activate the body's relaxation response, promoting a sense of calmness and reducing stress and anxiety levels. This relaxation response is vital for preparing the body and mind for sleep, as it helps to decrease the production of stress hormones such as cortisol, which can interfere with the ability to fall asleep and stay asleep throughout the night. Diaphragmatic breathing also facilitates better oxygen exchange in the body, leading to improved blood circulation and a decrease in muscle tension, which can further promote relaxation and induce sleepiness. Additionally, this technique can help individuals maintain a regular breathing pattern, which is essential for achieving a state of deep and restorative sleep. Incorporating diaphragmatic breathing into a nightly bedtime routine can thus serve as a natural and effective method for supporting overall sleep quality and enhancing relaxation.

Find a quiet place and sit in a comfortable position, with your knees bent and your shoulders, head and neck relaxed.
Place one hand on your upper chest and the other just below your rib cage. This will allow you to feel your diaphragm move as you breathe.
Breathe in slowly through your nose so that your stomach moves out against your hand. The hand on your chest should remain as still as possible.
Tighten your stomach muscles, letting them fall inward as you exhale through pursed lips. The hand on your upper chest must remain as still as possible.
We recommend that you start with 5-10 minutes, about 3-4 times per day. Gradually increase the amount of time you spend doing this exercise, and perhaps even increase the effort of the exercise by placing a book on your abdomen.

iii. MEDITATION

OVERVIEW

Meditation serves as a potent tool in fostering quality sleep by addressing both physiological and psychological factors that influence our ability to rest effectively.

Through consistent practice, meditation cultivates a state of relaxation and tranquility, helping to alleviate stress and anxiety, which are common inhibitors of sound sleep. By engaging in mindfulness meditation, individuals develop an enhanced awareness of their thoughts, emotions, and bodily sensations, enabling them to identify and manage sources of mental unrest that may disrupt sleep patterns. This heightened self-awareness facilitates the release of tension stored in the body, promoting physical relaxation conducive to falling asleep and staying asleep throughout the night.

Moreover, meditation techniques such as deep breathing exercises encourage the activation of the parasympathetic nervous system, which induces a state of calmness and promotes the body's natural transition into sleep mode. Additionally, regular meditation practices have been shown to regulate hormone levels, including cortisol and melatonin, which play crucial roles in the sleep-wake cycle. By modulating these hormonal responses, meditation can help regulate circadian rhythms and promote the onset of sleep at the appropriate time.

Furthermore, the cultivation of mindfulness through meditation enhances the ability to let go of intrusive thoughts and worries that may linger in the mind at bedtime, thus creating a mental environment conducive to falling asleep peacefully. Overall, meditation serves as a holistic approach to improving sleep quality by addressing the interconnectedness of mind and body, promoting relaxation, stress reduction, and fostering a deep sense of inner calm conducive to restful sleep.

CONCENTRATION MEDITATION

Concentration meditation, a practice rooted in focusing the mind on a single point of reference, offers a powerful avenue for enhancing and supporting quality sleep. By harnessing the ability to direct attention away from racing thoughts and distractions, concentration meditation promotes relaxation, reduces stress, and prepares the mind for restorative sleep.

Among the most popular techniques within concentration meditation is the "candle flame" method. Practitioners concentrate on the flame of a candle, allowing it to occupy their entire field of vision. As the mind becomes absorbed in the gentle flickering of the flame, other thoughts naturally recede, inducing a state of tranquility conducive to sleep. To apply concentration meditation effectively, one can start by finding a quiet space free from disturbances, assume a comfortable position, and focus entirely on the chosen point of concentration, whether it's the breath, a mantra, or an external object like the candle flame. With practice, this technique cultivates mental discipline, enhances relaxation

MINDFULNESS MEDITATION

Mindfulness meditation offers a powerful avenue for improving the quality of sleep by promoting relaxation and reducing stress and anxiety levels. One popular technique in mindfulness meditation for sleep is the body scan meditation. In this practice, individuals lie down comfortably and systematically direct their attention to different parts of their body, starting from the toes and gradually moving upward. By focusing on each part and noticing sensations without judgment, practitioners cultivate awareness of bodily tension and learn to release it, facilitating a state of deep relaxation conducive to sleep. Practical steps in applying mindfulness meditation for better sleep include finding a quiet, comfortable space, adopting a relaxed posture, and setting aside dedicated time each day for practice. Utilizing guided meditation recordings or apps can also aid beginners in staying focused and following along with the practice effectively.

Over time, you can become more aware of the human tendency to quickly judge an experience as good or bad, pleasant or unpleasant. With practice, an inner balance develops. In some schools of meditation, students practice a combination of concentration and mindfulness.
Many disciplines call for stillness and to a greater or lesser degree, depending on the teacher.

Some tips on how to meditate (example)
This exercise is an excellent introduction to a meditation technique.
Sit or lie comfortably.
Close your eyes.
Make no effort to control the breath and simply breathe naturally.
Focus your attention on the breath and on how the body moves with each inhalation and exhalation. Notice the movement of your body as you breathe.
Observe your chest, shoulders, rib cage, and belly. Simply focus your attention on your breath without controlling its pace or intensity.
If and when your mind wanders, return your focus back to your breath. Keep doing this.
Start with maintaining this meditation practice for five minutes and then try to extend for longer periods of time.
It is also very individual. Some prefer to include soothing sounds, or voices (guided meditation), or scents, or all of these and more. Others prefer none or total silence and isolation.
You need to consider what works best for you and will help you to get a good night's sleep.

iv. STRETCHING

Your muscles need activity for proper circulation and health, and if you're sitting hunched at your computer, or stressed out in traffic, your aching muscles will need some help at the end of the day to relax.

Stretching before bed is another great way to release tension from the day and get the best night's sleep.
Most people know to stretch before and after exercise, or in the morning to energise themselves, but there's actually a ton of reasons to stretch before bedtime as well.
In addition to getting regular exercise, stretching offers many benefits for our body and mind.

Developing an evening stretching routine helps our body enter a relaxed state quicker, and stay in a deeper sleep for longer. With fewer points of pain along your back, neck, and shoulders, we are less likely to toss and turn. This is great for not only our sleep, but also our partner's sleep, too.

Additionally, stretching does provide a great alternative nighttime activity to scrolling through social media or reading emails on a screen.
When done correctly, studies have shown that practices like yoga and stretching can be incredibly relaxing and meditative. Focusing on your body and the present actions can be a great way to separate yourself from the day's stresses and signal to your subconscious to stop worrying.

For some great examples of a stretching routine that will help relax your body, check out the stretches on Appendix A4.

v. POSTPONE YOUR WORRIES

As we mentioned in Chapter 2, "DURING DAYTIME" section, in our busy schedules, the first time we may have the opportunity to sit down and think is very often when we go to bed at night.

This is the worst time to start thinking as it often triggers arousal and leads to anxiety, therefore, it is highly recommended that a set time is scheduled during the day (ideally in the afternoon) to tackle any of the outstanding thoughts that pop up just before bedtime.
This is often referred to as "worry time". It is worth noting that "taking action" does not mean that you must resolve all issues there and then as some will most likely require more than 15 minutes. Coming up with an actionable plan and scheduling when that will be tackled may be just as sufficient during the "worry time" as the objective is to avoid these issues popping up before bedtime.
By learning to postpone your worries, it will be less intrusive before bedtime and will give you a greater sense of control.
It will require some persistence and patience to keep it going, yet it works well for most, so please give it a try.

It does take some time and patience as worry postponement may seem like a strange thing to do, and it may seem like an effort to jot down your worries and commit to sitting down and reflecting on the days worries at a set time everyday. Yet, it is important to do this at the start because it is a difficult and new skill you are developing. But with time and practice in this formal way, you will be able to do it effectively and more informally.
Also, typically people predict that they won't be able to postpone their worrying, but often people are surprised that they are actually able to postpone many of their worries, and experience a greater sense of control.
Below are three key steps to help you successfully achieve this.

STEP 1: set time for "worry time":
To begin, choose a particular time, place, and length of time for worrying. This time, place and duration should be the same each day, for example: 2pm, study room, 15 minutes. Make this place unique and comfortable, free from distractions. Ideally, it should not be somewhere you go regularly, like a lounge room chair, instead, it should be somewhere you allocate only for the "worry time".
The time should be convenient so you can regularly follow through with the task, time.

STEP 2: postpone your worries:
As part of the bedtime preparation, note down any outstanding actions that come to your mind. You can also do this any time of the day, or as soon as you become aware of such thoughts.

This activity will help you "postpone your worries" for a set time ("worry time") during the afternoon.

Here are some key steps:
• Note your worry briefly on paper (in a couple of words only).
• Remind yourself that you will have time to think about it later and that there is no need to worry about it now as you will be in a better position to deal with these during the scheduled "worry time".
• Remind yourself that there are more important or pleasant things to attend to right now, rather than worry.
• Turn your focus to the present moment and the activities of the day to help let go of the worry until the worry period has arrived.
• Decide what is the most important and best thing you can practically do for yourself right now. Take immediate action to do something that is either practical, positive, pleasant, active or nurturing.

STEP 3: time to tackle your worries ("worry time"):
Settle yourself down at the place you had planned and take some time to reflect on the worries you had written down from the day.

Some additional notes:
• Only worry about the things you have noted if you feel you must.
• If all or some of the worries you wrote down are no longer bothering you or no longer seem relevant, then no further action is required.
• If you do need to worry about some of them, spend no longer than the set amount of time you specified for your "worry time". It may also be helpful to write your thoughts on paper rather than worrying in your head. You can do this in whatever way feels right to you.

Please refer to Appendix 3 for a proposed approach to tackling "worry" items.

vi. OTHER METHODS

There are many various other methods and techniques to support getting quality sleep.

BATHING/SHOWERING (60 to 90 minutes before bed)

A nighttime bathing or showering may help send your brain the signal that it is time to sleep. Bathing or showering at night also ensures you will be cleaner when you go to bed, reducing the buildup of sweat, dirt, and body oils on your bedding.

A growing body of research suggests that taking a hot shower or bath before bed can improve sleep. In the hours before bedtime, a human's core body temperature naturally cools, while skin temperatures of the hands and feet increase. Scientists hypothesise that immersing the body in warm water aids this natural temperature regulation process, improving sleep as a result.

Warm water increases your circulation and draws heat from the core of your body to your fingers and toes. Then, when you step out of the bath or shower, your body cools in the air. It's this temperature drop that mimics one of the many cues our body uses to wind down.

When you're awake, your core body temperature is the highest, often in the late afternoon or early evening. This is part of your body's circadian rhythms, a set of behaviours and biochemistry timed to an internal 24-hour clock with a wake and sleep cycle. What triggers your sleep cycle is the natural decrease of body temperature, by roughly a degree, an hour before bedtime.

MASSAGE

Like bathing, massage is stimulating to your circulation and should generally be avoided immediately before bedtime. Prior to bedtime, however, try gently massaging your feet and legs with a calming massage oil or lotion.

TEA-TIME

Tea, especially herbal teas, using botanicals that have a natural sedative effect, which can be both soothing and relaxing before bedtime. A good example is a chamomile tea.

Teas made from passion flower and valerian are also considered to be very relaxing and help to encourage sleep, but do not have the familiar and pleasant flavour that chamomile tea offers.

GADGETS

Unfortunately, many of us consider our bedrooms as extensions of our living rooms and studies, and more than often introduce electronic devices (digital distractions) into our bedrooms.

As we already covered, the bedroom should be for sleeping only!

Electronic devices such as TVs, computers, smartphones and tablets are extremely disruptive and prevent us from falling asleep.

These devices also disrupt us during sleep, either noise from beeps and buzzes or lights from screens or flashing LEDs.

Therefore, it is highly recommended that we avoid bringing any electronics devices into our bedrooms or at least turn them off completely.

vii. OTHER RESOURCES

Please visit www.zeez.online for more information and material on the programme.

There is material for downloading, such as a:
- Three-Week Sleep Diary
- Sleep Questionnaire
- Bedtime Yoga

We plan to continue to add more material based on the feedback we receive.

And again, we would love to hear from you on your experience, such as, what has worked well, what could have been better and any other comments you may have. Please visit www.zeez.online to share your thoughts with us.

Thank you!

APPENDIX 1:
A1. Sleep Diary - Week 1:

INTRODUCTION:
1. The Sleep Diary must be completed in the morning, for example, Day 1 is the first morning.

2. The Sleep Diary is „more art than science" therefore it is important to take notes, with emphasis on capturing records as estimates as oppose to precise answers.

3. It is essential to capture the highlights from each week, such as what worked well and what could have been better.

4. You can download the entire three-week programme from https://www.zeez.online, DOWNLOADS section.

APPENDIX 1 (cont.):
A1. Sleep Diary - Table Week 1:

	Day 1	Day 2	Day 3	Day 4	Day 5	Day 6	Day 7
What time did you go to bed last night?							
How long did it take you to fall asleep?							
How many times did you wake up in the night?							
For how long were you awake during the night in total?							
At what time did you finally wake up?							
At what time did you get up?							
How long did you spend in bed last night?							
Please rate (scale from 1 - 10) the quality of your sleep from last night? (1=low, 10=high)							

APPENDIX 1 (cont.):
A1. Sleep Diary - Table Week 2:

	Day 1	Day 2	Day 3	Day 4	Day 5	Day 6	Day 7
What time did you go to bed last night?							
How long did it take you to fall asleep?							
How many times did you wake up in the night?							
For how long were you awake during the night in total?							
At what time did you finally wake up?							
At what time did you get up?							
How long did you spend in bed last night?							
Please rate (scale from 1 - 10) the quality of your sleep from last night? (1=low, 10=high)							

APPENDIX 1 (cont.):
A1. Sleep Diary - Table Week 3:

	Day 1	Day 2	Day 3	Day 4	Day 5	Day 6	Day 7
What time did you go to bed last night?							
How long did it take you to fall asleep?							
How many times did you wake up in the night?							
For how long were you awake during the night in total?							
At what time did you finally wake up?							
At what time did you get up?							
How long did you spend in bed last night?							
Please rate (scale from 1 - 10) the quality of your sleep from last night? (1=low, 10=high)							

APPENDIX 2:
A2. Sleep Questionnaire – Ranking Intro

INTRODUCTION:
The following questions can be helpful to capture the current and broader states of sleep. These can also provide indications of areas of potential disorders.
It is best when the questionnaire is completed at the start of the programme and again at the end to highlight progress and potential gaps to be further addressed.
See guide notes below.

Also, you can download the entire questionnaire from DOWNLOADS section: https://www.zeez.online.

GUIDE NOTES:
Please note that this should not serve as a substitute for any clinical evaluation. For a more detailed clinical evaluation you must refer to a medical professional or professional psychology specialist.

1. Ranking of 3, 4 or 5 on any question generally indicates sleep disorders, including insomnia.
Also rankings of 3, 4 or 5 on any question, for two or more questions generally indicates some form of daytime impairment and may require further evaluation.

2. Ranking of 4 or 5 on questions 6 and/or 7 are likely to indicate symptoms of insomnia or non-restorative sleep.

APPENDIX 2 (cont.):
A2. Sleep Questionnaire – Ranking Intro

3. Ranking of 4 or 5 on questions 9 and/or 10 are likely to indicate that you may require further clinical evaluation for sleep apnea.

4. Ranking of 4 or 5 on questions 11 is likely to indicate a circadian rhythm disorder. Further questioning about shift work or a preference for a delayed sleep phase should be done.

APPENDIX 2 (cont.):
A2. Sleep Questionnaire – Ranking Table

	Never	Occasionally / Rarely	Neutral	Frequently / Often	Always
Do you have trouble falling asleep?					
Do you have trouble staying asleep?					
Do you take anything to help you sleep?					
Do you use alcohol to help you sleep?					
Do you use any medication to help you sleep?					
Are your legs restless and/or uncomfortable before bed?					
Do you have any unusual behaviours or movements during sleep?					
Do you have difficulty staying awake during the day?					
Do you snore?					
Has anyone said that you stop breathing, gasp, snort, or choke in your sleep?					
Are you a shift worker or is your sleep schedule irregular?					

APPENDIX 3:
A3. Tackling worries ("worry time tree")

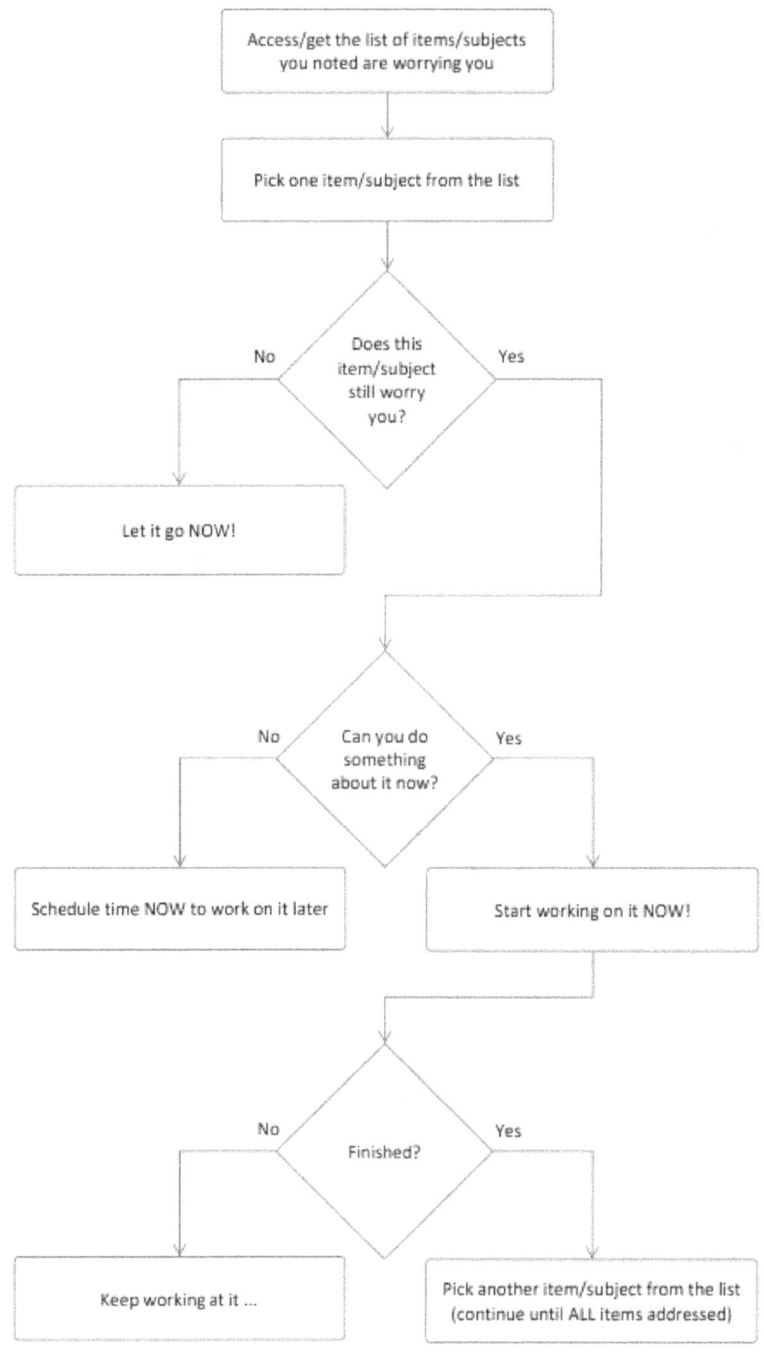

APPENDIX 4:
A4. Stretching (provided by Ocean Moon Yoga)

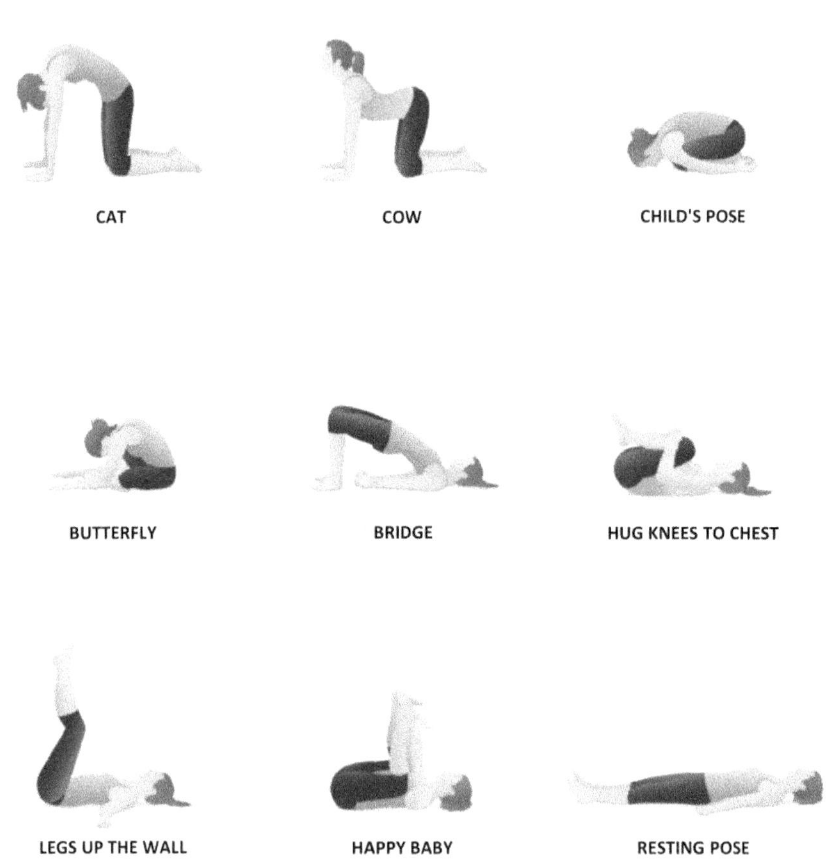

source: https://www.oceanmoonyoga.com

APPENDIX 5:
Sleep Hygiene Checklist – Top 12 items

1. Maintain a consistent sleep schedule, going to bed and waking up at the same time every day.

2. Create a relaxing bedtime routine to signal your body that it's time to sleep.

3. Make sure your sleep environment is dark, quiet, and cool.

4. Use your bed only for sleep and intimacy, avoiding activities like work or watching TV in bed.

5. Avoid consuming stimulants like caffeine and nicotine close to bedtime.

6. Limit exposure to electronic devices, such as smartphones and tablets, before bed.

7. Engage in regular physical activity during the day, but avoid intense exercise close to bedtime.

8. Avoid large meals, spicy foods, and excessive fluid intake before bedtime.

9. Create a comfortable and supportive sleep surface with a good-quality mattress and pillows.

10. Manage stress through relaxation techniques, such as deep breathing or meditation.

11. Avoid napping during the day, especially in the late afternoon or evening.

12. Limit alcohol consumption, as it can disrupt sleep patterns.

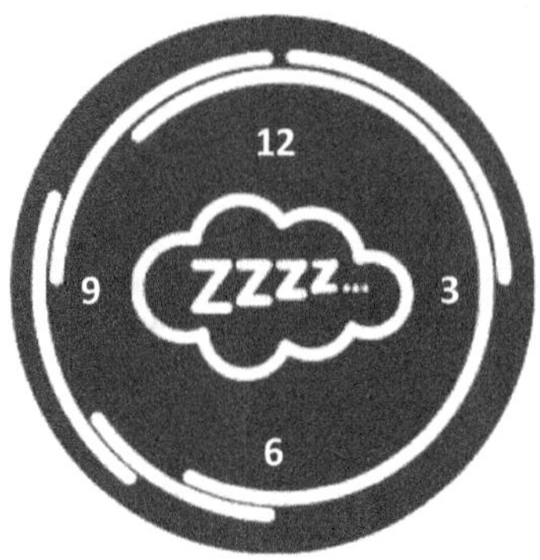

visit us on: https://www.zeez.online